I0695850

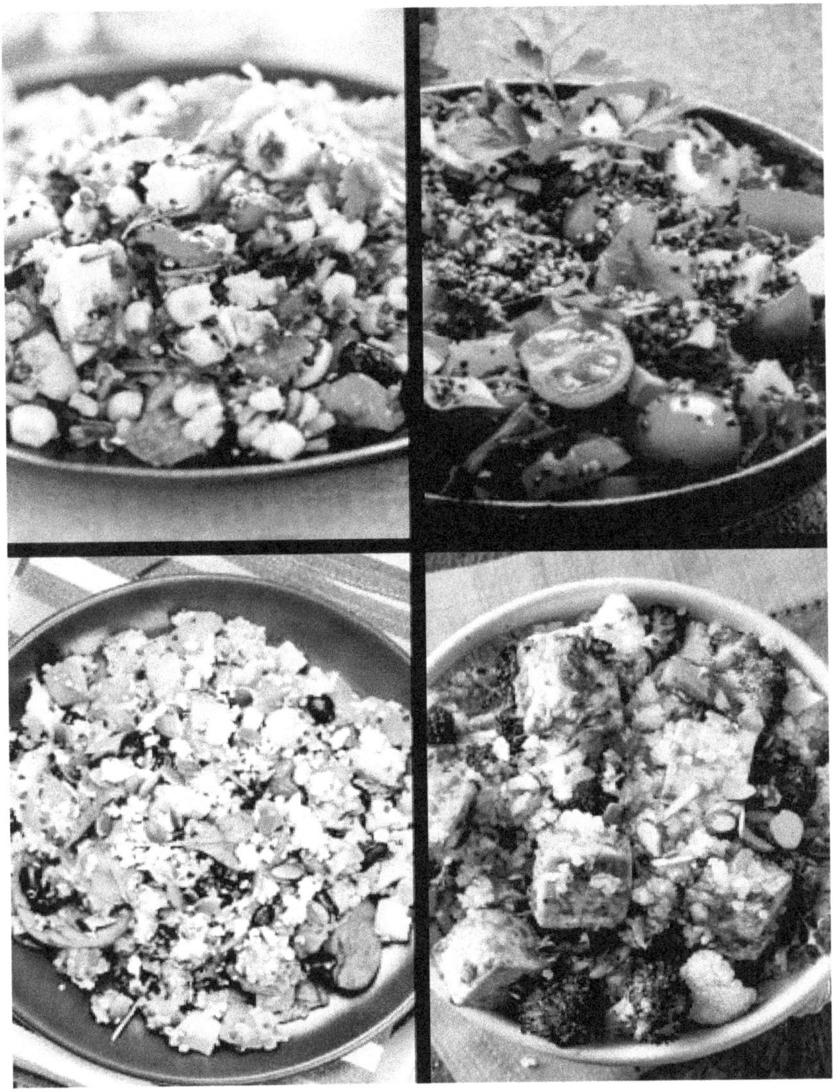

THE GALVESTON DIET MEAL PLAN

Unlocking Hormonal Balance for Lasting Weight Loss

By

DR. MURIEL JORDAN

Copyright (c) 2023 by Dr. Muriel Jordan

The information contained in this book is based on the best available sources at the time of writing. The author and the publisher make no warranties or representations, express or implied, with respect to the accuracy or completeness of the contents of this book and specifically disclaim any implied warranties of merchantability or fitness for a particular purpose. The author and publisher shall not be held liable for any loss or damages whatsoever arising from, or in connection with, the use of this book.

This book is intended for informational purposes only. The author and publisher do not offer any medical, legal, or professional advice. If you require such advice, please seek the services of a competent professional.

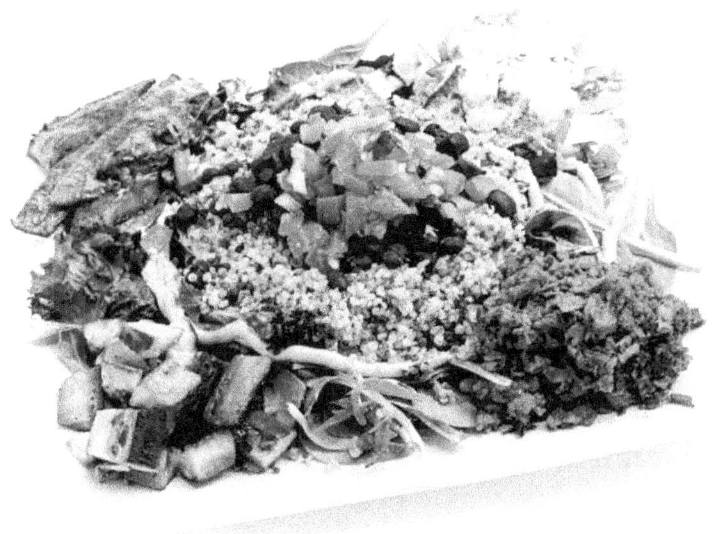

Table of contents

Introduction

Welcome to "The Galveston Diet Meal Plan," a comprehensive guide that promises to revolutionize your approach to wellness and weight management. In a world inundated with fleeting health trends, this journey offers something different—a profound understanding of how hormones, nutrition, and lifestyle choices intertwine to shape our bodies and lives.

Through the chapters that follow, we will embark on an exploration of the intricate relationship between hormones and weight gain. The Galveston Diet recognizes that hormones play a pivotal role in our overall health, particularly in the context of weight management. By unraveling the roles of hormones such as insulin, cortisol, and estrogen, we gain insights into the mechanisms that influence weight gain and learn how to harness these physiological forces to our advantage.

At the heart of the Galveston Diet philosophy lies a set of fundamental principles that guide us toward optimal well-being. In the chapter dedicated to these principles, we will uncover the wisdom of balanced nutrition, mindful eating, and strategic meal planning. This holistic approach not only supports weight loss but also fosters a harmonious relationship with food, empowering us to make conscious choices that nourish both body and soul.

Intermittent fasting, a time-tested practice, assumes a central role within the Galveston Diet strategy. In a world where constant consumption is the norm, embracing periods of controlled fasting can reset our metabolic processes, enhance hormone sensitivity, and accelerate progress toward our weight management goals. In the chapter on intermittent fasting, we will explore the science behind this approach and provide practical guidance on integrating it into your daily routine.

Transitioning to the practical realm, we present a meticulously crafted Galveston Diet meal plan encompassing breakfast, lunch, and dinner. These nourishing and flavorful meals are designed to fuel your body, delight your taste buds, and align with the diet's principles. With a diverse array of options, mealtime becomes a celebration of both health and culinary pleasure.

Physical activity is not just a means to burn calories; it's a gateway to holistic well-being. The Galveston Diet recognizes the significance of movement and exercise in achieving optimal health. In the chapter dedicated to exercise and motion, you'll discover how to infuse your routine with enjoyable physical activities that elevate your energy, enhance your mood, and complement your weight management efforts.

Beyond nutrition and physical activity, stress control and sleep enhancement emerge as crucial pillars of the Galveston Diet. Managing stress and prioritizing restorative sleep is integral to hormonal balance and overall well-being. In this section, we explore strategies to cultivate inner serenity, navigate stressors, and foster healthy sleep patterns.

Women traversing the transformative phase of menopause will find tailored guidance in the Galveston Diet strategy.

Menopause brings unique hormonal shifts that can impact weight and well-being. Our guide provides insights into managing these changes through nutrition, lifestyle adjustments, and self-care, empowering women to embrace this phase with resilience and vitality.

The culmination of this journey leads us to sustained weight management—the ultimate goal of the Galveston Diet. Armed with a deep understanding of hormones, nutrition, and lifestyle dynamics, you'll be equipped to maintain your progress, make informed choices, and embrace the Galveston Diet as a lifelong companion on your wellness voyage.

In "The Galveston Diet Meal Plan," knowledge merges with empowerment to create a transformative roadmap for vibrant health. Join us as we unlock the secrets of hormonal balance, embrace mindful nourishment, and forge a path toward enduring well-being. This is not merely a diet; it's a holistic lifestyle shift that celebrates the innate wisdom of your body and empowers you to create a future brimming with vitality.

Chapter 1

Hormones and Their Impact on Weight Gain

Hormones, the intricate messengers of our body, orchestrate a symphony of physiological processes that influence our overall health and well-being. Among their multifaceted roles, hormones hold a prominent place in regulating weight gain and body composition. The delicate balance of these chemical messengers can significantly impact our metabolism, appetite, fat storage, and energy expenditure. In this exploration, we delve into the fascinating world of hormones and their profound influence on weight gain.

Insulin: The Blood Sugar Regulator

One of the most well-known hormones associated with weight gain is insulin. Produced by the pancreas, insulin plays a crucial role in maintaining blood sugar levels. When we ingest carbohydrates, they undergo a process of breakdown into glucose, leading to a rise in blood sugar levels. Insulin is then released to facilitate the uptake of glucose into cells, where it is used for energy or stored as glycogen in the liver and muscles. However, in the presence of consistently high blood sugar levels, often a result of excessive carbohydrate consumption, insulin promotes the storage of excess glucose as fat. This process, especially prevalent in conditions like insulin resistance, contributes to weight gain and obesity.

Leptin: The Satiety Signal

Leptin, often referred to as the "satiety hormone," is produced by fat cells and acts as a communicator between the body's fat stores and the brain. Its primary role is to signal the brain when sufficient energy stores are available, effectively curbing appetite and promoting energy expenditure. In cases of obesity, the body may become resistant to the effects of leptin, leading to a disruption in this satiety signaling pathway. As a result, individuals may overeat due to a lack of perceived fullness, contributing to further weight gain.

Ghrelin: The Hunger Hormone

On the other side of the appetite spectrum, ghrelin, often referred to as the "hunger hormone," stimulates appetite and encourages food intake. Produced mainly in the stomach, ghrelin levels increase before meals and decrease after eating. However, hormonal imbalances or disrupted meal patterns can lead to higher ghrelin levels, potentially driving individuals to consume more calories than needed. This overconsumption, if sustained, can lead to weight gain over time.

Cortisol: Stress and Weight

The stress hormone cortisol, produced by the adrenal glands, is a vital component of the body's fight-or-flight response. While crucial in short bursts, chronic stress can lead to persistently elevated cortisol levels. This chronic stress response has been linked to weight gain, particularly in the abdominal region. Cortisol increases appetite and encourages the storage of fat, especially visceral fat, which surrounds internal organs and poses a higher risk of metabolic complications.

Thyroid Hormones: Metabolic Conductors

Thyroid hormones, primarily thyroxine (T4) and triiodothyronine (T3) play a central role in regulating metabolism. These hormones influence the rate at which the body expends energy and processes nutrients. An underactive thyroid (hypothyroidism) can slow down metabolism, leading to weight gain, fatigue, and other related symptoms. Conversely, an overactive thyroid (hyperthyroidism) can accelerate metabolism, causing weight loss, rapid heartbeat, and nervousness.

Sex Hormones: Estrogen and Testosterone

The influence of sex hormones extends beyond reproduction, impacting weight regulation as well. Estrogen, predominantly produced in the ovaries, has been shown to influence fat distribution. During menopause, when estrogen levels decline, there is a shift in fat storage from the hips and thighs to the abdomen. This change in fat distribution is associated with increased risk factors for cardiovascular disease and insulin resistance. In males, reduced testosterone levels can contribute to increased fat mass and decreased muscle mass, potentially leading to weight gain.

Hormonal Disorders and Weight Gain

Certain hormonal disorders can directly contribute to weight gain. Polycystic ovary syndrome (PCOS), a common endocrine disorder in women, is characterized by insulin resistance and hormonal imbalances. Insulin resistance associated with PCOS can lead to increased fat storage, particularly around the abdomen. Additionally, hormonal treatments, such as corticosteroids or certain medications, may also influence weight gain as a side effect.

Managing Hormonal Impact on Weight Gain

Understanding the intricate relationship between hormones and weight gain is pivotal in developing effective strategies for weight management. Lifestyle modifications are a cornerstone of hormonal balance. A balanced diet that supports stable blood sugar levels, incorporating whole grains, lean proteins, healthy fats, and ample fruits and vegetables, can help regulate insulin and prevent excessive fat storage. Regular physical activity enhances insulin sensitivity and supports weight management by promoting calorie expenditure.

Stress management techniques, such as mindfulness, meditation, and relaxation exercises, can mitigate the effects of cortisol on weight gain. Prioritizing adequate sleep is also crucial, as sleep deprivation can disrupt hormonal balance and lead to increased appetite and weight gain.

Individualized approaches, considering hormonal status, can be beneficial. For instance, individuals with PCOS may benefit from dietary changes that manage insulin resistance. Medical interventions, such as hormone replacement therapy for menopause-related weight gain, may be considered under the guidance of healthcare professionals.

Hormones wield remarkable influence over our body's intricate systems, including weight regulation. The complex interplay between insulin, leptin, ghrelin, cortisol, thyroid hormones, and sex hormones orchestrates our metabolic dance. While hormones can impact weight gain, they are not the sole determinants. Lifestyle choices, including diet, exercise, stress management, and sleep, play an integral role in maintaining hormonal balance and achieving a healthy weight. By understanding the role of hormones and adopting a holistic approach to health, we empower ourselves to navigate the dynamic world of weight management with knowledge and resilience.

Chapter 2

The Galveston Diet: Fundamental Principles and Recommendations

In the realm of dietary approaches aimed at enhancing health and managing weight, the Galveston Diet stands out for its focus on hormonal equilibrium and personalized well-being. This method, centered around addressing hormonal changes, particularly in women aged 40 and above, offers a unique perspective on dietary habits. In this chapter, we delve into the core principles and recommendations that define the Galveston Diet.

Understanding Hormones and Weight Management

As individuals age, hormonal fluctuations can significantly impact various aspects of their lives, including metabolism, energy levels, and body composition. These hormonal changes, most notably during perimenopause and menopause, can contribute to weight gain, alterations in fat storage, and changes in body structure. The Galveston Diet recognizes the critical role that hormones play in these processes and seeks to restore equilibrium through strategic dietary choices.

The Foundation of the Galveston Diet

Central to the Galveston Diet are the principles of intermittent fasting and carbohydrate cycling. Intermittent fasting involves cycling between periods of eating and fasting, allowing the body to utilize stored fat for energy during fasting intervals. This process aids in weight loss while preserving lean muscle mass. Carbohydrate cycling, on the other hand, entails altering carbohydrate intake levels throughout the week to align with the body's natural hormonal rhythms.

Key Principles and Recommendations

Intermittent Fasting: The Galveston Diet encourages a 16:8 fasting protocol, which translates to fasting for 16 hours and consuming meals within an 8-hour timeframe. This fasting approach is designed to promote fat oxidation and enhance insulin sensitivity. Delaying the first meal of the day can contribute to achieving the fasting window.

Carbohydrate Cycling: The diet advocates for a variation in carbohydrate consumption, with higher carbohydrate intake on certain days and reduced intake on others. This strategy is aligned with hormonal fluctuations, utilizing higher-carb days to support thyroid function and optimize insulin sensitivity.

Nutrient-Dense Foods: Prioritizing nutrient-dense whole foods forms a core aspect of the Galveston Diet. This entails incorporating lean proteins, a diverse range of vegetables and fruits, whole grains, and healthy fats. Such foods offer essential vitamins, minerals, and antioxidants that contribute to overall health and hormonal balance.

Hydration: Adequate hydration remains a fundamental aspect of hormonal balance and well-being. The Galveston Diet recommends consuming ample water, herbal teas, and other hydrating beverages throughout the day.

Limit Processed Foods: Processed foods that are high in refined sugars, unhealthy fats, and artificial additives can disrupt hormonal equilibrium and contribute to weight gain. The diet advises minimizing the intake of such foods to promote optimal health.

Exercise and Movement: Regular physical activity is integral to the Galveston Diet. A balanced routine that includes both cardiovascular exercise and strength training can boost metabolism, preserve lean muscle mass, and contribute to achieving weight-related objectives.

Stress Management: Recognizing the influence of stress on hormones and weight gain, the diet suggests incorporating stress management techniques into daily life. Meditation, deep breathing exercises, and mindfulness practices can mitigate the impact of stress on hormonal balance.

Personalization: Acknowledging the uniqueness of each individual's hormonal profile and metabolism, the Galveston Diet advocates for a personalized approach. By paying attention to cues from the body and making adjustments based on energy levels and hunger signals, individuals can fine-tune their fasting and carbohydrate cycling patterns.

Scientific Basis and Considerations

While the Galveston Diet provides a tailored approach to weight management, it's important to note that its principles may not be universally supported by the scientific community. Some experts and healthcare professionals raise questions about the necessity of carbohydrate cycling and the variability of benefits associated with intermittent fasting.

The diet's focus on hormonal balance is grounded in the understanding that hormones contribute to weight dynamics. However, critics emphasize that the relationship between hormones and weight gain is intricate, with factors such as genetics, lifestyle, and overall health playing pivotal roles.

Practical Implementation and Conclusion

Before embarking on any dietary plan, consulting a healthcare professional is recommended, particularly for those with underlying health conditions or specific dietary requirements. Here are some practical considerations for individuals interested in adopting the Galveston Diet:

Consultation: Seek guidance from a healthcare provider or registered dietitian to determine the compatibility of the Galveston Diet with your health objectives and individual needs.

Gradual Transition: If new to intermittent fasting or carbohydrate cycling, ease into these practices gradually to allow your body to adapt.

Diverse and Balanced Diet: Ensure that your diet encompasses a variety of nutrient-rich foods to fulfill your nutritional requirements.

Body Awareness: Pay attention to your body's responses to fasting and carbohydrate cycling. Make adjustments as needed to sustain energy levels and overall well-being.

Comprehensive Approach: Remember that diet is just one facet of overall health. Prioritize adequate sleep, stress management, and regular physical activity to support holistic well-being.

The Galveston Diet introduces a distinctive angle to weight management by emphasizing hormonal equilibrium through intermittent fasting and carbohydrate cycling. As with any dietary approach, critical thinking and an understanding of individual variability are crucial. While the Galveston Diet may not be suitable for everyone, seeking guidance from healthcare professionals and integrating scientific evidence can pave the way for a more comprehensive and personalized approach to health and wellness.

Chapter 3

Intermittent Fasting within the Galveston Nutritional Strategy

In the ever-evolving landscape of dietary approaches, one methodology that has garnered significant attention is intermittent fasting . When integrated into the Galveston Nutritional Strategy, intermittent fasting takes on a distinctive role in harnessing the potential of hormonal balance and personalized well-being. This comprehensive exploration delves into the core principles, mechanisms, benefits, and considerations of intermittent fasting within the Galveston Nutritional Strategy.

Understanding Intermittent Fasting

Intermittent fasting involves cycling between periods of eating and fasting, where individuals abstain from consuming calories for designated intervals. It is important to note that intermittent fasting is not about restricting the types of foods one eats, but rather focuses on the timing of meals. This practice prompts the body to tap into its energy reserves, particularly stored fat, during fasting periods, resulting in potential weight loss and other health benefits.

Intermittent Fasting in the Context of the Galveston Nutritional Strategy

The Galveston Nutritional Strategy is underpinned by the recognition of hormonal fluctuations and their profound influence on weight management, particularly in women over the age of 40. This unique approach capitalizes on the concept of intermittent fasting to leverage hormonal balance and support overall well-being.

The Fundamental Principles of Intermittent Fasting in the Galveston Nutritional Strategy

Time-Restricted Eating Window: Central to the Galveston Nutritional Strategy is the concept of a time-restricted eating window. This window typically follows a 16:8 fasting protocol, where individuals fast for 16 hours and consume their meals within an 8-hour timeframe. By limiting the eating window, the body has an extended period to access stored energy, potentially leading to weight loss and improved metabolic efficiency.

Optimization of Hormonal Balance: Intermittent fasting aligns harmoniously with the Galveston Nutritional Strategy's emphasis on hormonal equilibrium. As the fasting periods encourage the body to rely on stored fat for energy, insulin sensitivity may improve. This can play a pivotal role in addressing insulin resistance, a hallmark of hormonal imbalance that can contribute to weight gain.

Enhancement of Fat Oxidation: During fasting periods, insulin levels decline, signaling the body to shift from using glucose for energy to utilizing stored fat. This increased fat oxidation can contribute to weight loss and promote a leaner body composition.

Mechanisms Underlying Intermittent Fasting

The benefits of intermittent fasting within the Galveston Nutritional Strategy are rooted in several intricate mechanisms:

Insulin Sensitivity: Intermittent fasting may enhance insulin sensitivity, making cells more responsive to insulin's actions. This can help regulate blood sugar levels and reduce the risk of insulin resistance, a condition linked to weight gain and hormonal imbalances.

Autophagy: Fasting triggers a process known as autophagy, which involves the removal of damaged or dysfunctional cellular components. This cellular "clean-up" process can support overall cellular health and potentially contribute to longevity.

Hormonal Regulation: Intermittent fasting has been shown to influence the secretion of hormones related to hunger and satiety, such as ghrelin and leptin. This can help individuals better manage their appetite and reduce overeating.

Metabolic Flexibility: Regular intermittent fasting can promote metabolic flexibility, allowing the body to seamlessly switch between using glucose and stored fat for energy. This adaptability can enhance overall metabolic efficiency.

Benefits of Intermittent Fasting within the Galveston Nutritional Strategy

Weight Management: One of the most notable benefits of intermittent fasting is its potential to support weight loss and weight maintenance. By creating a calorie deficit during fasting periods, individuals may experience a reduction in overall calorie intake, leading to weight loss over time.

Hormonal Balance: Intermittent fasting can contribute to hormonal balance by improving insulin sensitivity and reducing insulin resistance. This can be particularly advantageous in addressing hormonal fluctuations commonly observed in perimenopausal and menopausal women.

Cardiovascular Health: Research suggests that intermittent fasting may improve markers of cardiovascular health, including blood pressure, cholesterol levels, and triglycerides. These improvements can reduce the risk of cardiovascular diseases.

Cognitive Function: Intermittent fasting has been associated with potential cognitive benefits, such as improved brain health, enhanced focus, and reduced risk of neurodegenerative conditions. These effects may be attributed to increased production of brain-derived neurotrophic factor

(BDNF), a protein that supports brain function.

Inflammation Reduction: Chronic inflammation is linked to various health issues, including obesity and metabolic disorders. Intermittent fasting may help reduce inflammation markers in the body, contributing to improved overall health.

Considerations and Practical Implementation

While intermittent fasting offers a range of potential benefits, its implementation within the Galveston Nutritional Strategy requires careful consideration:

Personalization: As with any dietary approach, individual needs and preferences vary. Some individuals may find a 16:8 fasting protocol suitable, while others may prefer different fasting intervals. Personalization is key to optimizing the benefits of intermittent fasting.

Gradual Transition: For those new to intermittent fasting, a gradual transition is advised. Start by extending the fasting window gradually and paying attention to how your body responds.

Nutrient Density: During eating windows, prioritize nutrient-dense foods to meet your nutritional requirements. A balanced intake of protein, healthy fats, and a variety of fruits and vegetables supports overall well-being.

Hydration: Stay hydrated during fasting periods by consuming water, herbal teas, and other non-caloric beverages.

Listening to Your Body: It's crucial to listen to your body's cues. If you experience fatigue, dizziness, or discomfort during fasting periods, adjust your fasting approach accordingly.

Intermittent fasting, skillfully integrated within the Galveston Nutritional Strategy, presents a dynamic and personalized approach to weight management and hormonal balance. By harnessing the body's innate capacity to adapt to fasting periods, individuals can potentially experience weight loss, improved insulin sensitivity, and enhanced overall well-being. As with any dietary approach, individual consultation, thoughtful implementation, and ongoing adjustments are key to reaping the benefits of intermittent fasting within the context of the Galveston Nutritional Strategy. Through a harmonious synergy of hormonal equilibrium and dietary choices, individuals can embark on a journey toward sustainable health and vitality.

Chapter 4

The Galveston Diet Meal Plan for Breakfast

The Galveston Diet breakfast meal plan is designed to kickstart your day with nutrient-dense choices that promote hormonal balance and sustained energy. By focusing on a combination of lean proteins, healthy fats, and fiber-rich carbohydrates, the breakfast options support your body's natural rhythms and contribute to overall well-being.

1. Scrambled Eggs with Spinach and Avocado

Ingredients:

- 2 large eggs

- 1 cup fresh spinach, chopped

- 1/4 avocado, sliced

- Salt and pepper to taste

- Cooking spray or olive oil

Preparation:

1. Warm a non-stick skillet over medium heat and gently apply a thin layer of cooking spray or olive oil.

2. In a separate bowl, beat the eggs together with a dash of salt and pepper.

3. Pour the whisked eggs into the skillet and add chopped spinach.

4. Scramble the eggs and spinach until cooked to your preference.

5. Serve with avocado slices on top.

2. Greek Yogurt Parfait with Nuts and Berries

Ingredients:

- 1/2 cup Greek yogurt

- 1/4 cup mixed berries (e.g., blueberries, strawberries, raspberries)

- 1 tablespoon chia seeds

- 1 tablespoon chopped nuts (e.g., almonds, walnuts)

- 1 teaspoon honey (optional)

Preparation:

1. In a glass or bowl, layer Greek yogurt, mixed berries, chia seeds, and chopped nuts.

2. Drizzle honey over the top, if desired.

3. Enjoy this nutrient-packed parfait.

3. Veggie Omelette with Sautéed Mushrooms and Bell Peppers

Ingredients:

- 3 large eggs

- 1/4 cup sliced mushrooms

- 1/4 cup diced bell peppers

- 1/4 cup diced onions

- Salt and pepper to taste

- Cooking spray or olive oil

Preparation:

1. Heat a non-stick skillet over medium heat and coat with cooking spray or olive oil.

2. Sauté mushrooms, bell peppers, and onions until tender.

3. Combine the eggs with salt and pepper, whisking them in a bowl.

4. Pour the whisked eggs into the skillet, covering the sautéed veggies.

5. Continue cooking until the eggs firm up, then proceed to fold the omelette in half.

6. Serve with a side of fresh salsa or avocado slices.

4. Overnight Chia Pudding with Almond Butter and Berries

Ingredients:

- 2 tablespoons chia seeds

- 1/2 cup unsweetened almond milk

- 1 tablespoon almond butter

- 1/4 cup mixed berries

- 1 teaspoon honey (optional)

Preparation:

1. In a container or jar, mix together chia seeds and almond milk. Ensure thorough stirring.

2. Refrigerate overnight or for at least 4 hours until the mixture thickens.

3. Before serving, stir in almond butter and top with mixed berries.

4. Drizzle honey over the top, if desired.

5. Quinoa Breakfast Bowl with Fruit and Nuts

Ingredients:

- 1/2 cup cooked quinoa

- 1/4 cup Greek yogurt

- 1/4 cup mixed fresh fruit (e.g., mango, kiwi, berries)

- 1 tablespoon chopped nuts (e.g., pistachios, cashews)

- 1 teaspoon honey (optional)

Preparation:

1. In a bowl, layer cooked quinoa, Greek yogurt, and mixed fresh fruit.

2. Top with chopped nuts and drizzle with honey, if desired.

3. A satisfying and nutrient-rich breakfast bowl is ready to enjoy.

6. Spinach and Mushroom Frittata

Ingredients:

- 4 large eggs

- 1 cup fresh spinach, chopped

- 1/2 cup sliced mushrooms

- 1/4 cup diced onions

- Salt and pepper to taste

- Cooking spray or olive oil

Preparation:

1. Preheat the oven to 350°F (175°C).

2. In a bowl, whisk the eggs with pepper and salt.

3. Heat an oven-safe skillet over medium heat, and coat with cooking spray or olive oil.

4. Sauté mushrooms and onions until softened, then add chopped spinach.

5. Pour the whisked eggs over the sautéed veggies in the skillet.

6. Cook on the stovetop for a few minutes, then transfer the skillet to the preheated oven.

7. Place in the oven and bake for around 10 to 15 minutes, or until the frittata has fully solidified.

8. Slice and serve with a side of fresh salad.

7. Berry Protein Smoothie Bowl

Ingredients:

- 1/2 cup assorted berries (such as blueberries, strawberries, and raspberries)

- 1/2 banana

- 1 scoop protein powder (plant-based or whey)

- 1/2 cup unsweetened almond milk

- Toppings: sliced banana, chia seeds, granola

Preparation:

1. In a blender, combine mixed berries, bananas, protein powder, and almond milk.

2. Blend until smooth and creamy.

3. Transfer the smoothie to a bowl and garnish it with banana slices, chia seeds, and granola on top.

8. Avocado and Tomato Breakfast Salad

Ingredients:

- 1 avocado, diced

- 1 cup cherry tomatoes, halved

- 1/4 cup diced red onion

- Fresh basil leaves, torn

- Olive oil and balsamic vinegar for dressing

- Salt and pepper to taste

Preparation:

1. In a bowl, combine diced avocado, cherry tomatoes, and red onion.

2. Drizzle with olive oil and balsamic vinegar.

3. Season with salt and pepper, then top with torn basil leaves.

9. Nut Butter and Banana Wrap

Ingredients:

- 1 whole-grain tortilla or wrap

- 2 tablespoons almond butter or peanut butter

- 1 banana, sliced

- Cinnamon for sprinkling

Preparation:

1. Spread almond butter or peanut butter on the tortilla.

2. Place sliced banana on one side of the tortilla.

3. Sprinkle cinnamon over the banana slices.

4. Wrap the tortilla and relish a fulfilling breakfast wrap.

10. Vegetable Breakfast Stir-Fry

Ingredients:

- 2 eggs, beaten

- 1 cup mixed vegetables (e.g., bell peppers, zucchini, broccoli)

- 1/4 cup diced onions

- 1 teaspoon low-sodium soy sauce or tamari

- 1 teaspoon sesame oil

- Cooking spray or olive oil

Preparation:

1. Heat a non-stick skillet over medium heat and coat with cooking spray or olive oil.

2. Sauté diced onions and mixed vegetables until tender.

3. Push the vegetables to the side of the skillet and pour the beaten eggs into the empty space.

4. Scramble the eggs and combine them with the sautéed vegetables.

5. Drizzle with low-sodium soy sauce or tamari and sesame oil.

6. Stir-fry until heated through and well combined.

The Galveston Diet breakfast meal plan offers a diverse range of delicious options that align with the principles of hormone balance and overall wellness. By incorporating these nutrient-packed recipes into your morning routine, you set the stage for a day filled with nourishment and vitality. Whether you prefer eggs, yogurt, smoothies, or whole grains, the Galveston Diet breakfast recipes provide a balanced start to support your health and well-being journey.

Chapter 5

The Galveston Diet Meal Plan For Lunch

The Galveston Diet lunch meal plan is designed to provide a satisfying and nutrient-dense midday meal that supports hormonal balance and overall wellness. By focusing on a combination of lean proteins, fiber-rich carbohydrates, and healthy fats, these lunch options contribute to stable energy levels and promote a sense of vitality throughout the day.

1. Grilled Chicken and Quinoa Salad

Ingredients:

- 4 oz grilled chicken breast

- 1 cup cooked quinoa

- Mixed salad greens

- Cherry tomatoes, halved

- Cucumber slices

- Red onion, thinly sliced

- Olive oil and balsamic vinegar dressing

Preparation:

1. Grill the chicken breast and slice it.

2. In a bowl, combine quinoa, mixed greens, cherry tomatoes, cucumber, and red onion.

3. Top with sliced chicken and drizzle with olive oil and balsamic vinegar dressing.

2. Lentil and Vegetable Soup

Ingredients:

- 1 cup cooked green lentils

- Mixed vegetables (carrots, celery, zucchini)

- Low-sodium vegetable broth

- Garlic and onion, minced

- Fresh herbs (thyme, rosemary)

- Salt and pepper to taste

Preparation:

1. In a saucepan, cook garlic and onion until they release a pleasant aroma.

2. Add mixed vegetables, lentils, and vegetable broth.

3. Simmer until vegetables are tender, then season with fresh herbs, salt, and pepper.

3. Salmon and Asparagus with Quinoa

Ingredients:

- 4 oz baked or grilled salmon fillet

- Asparagus spears, trimmed

- 1 cup cooked quinoa

- Lemon juice and zest

- Fresh dill

- Olive oil

Preparation:

1. Bake or grill the salmon fillet and set aside.

2. Roast asparagus with a drizzle of olive oil.

3. Serve the salmon and asparagus over quinoa, drizzled with lemon juice and zest, and garnish with fresh dill.

4. Chickpea and Vegetable Stir-Fry

Ingredients:

- 1 cup cooked chickpeas

- Mixed vegetables (bell peppers, broccoli, snap peas)

- Low-sodium soy sauce or tamari

- Garlic and ginger, minced

- Sesame oil

- Cooked brown rice

Preparation:

1. Sauté garlic and ginger in sesame oil.

2. Add mixed vegetables and cooked chickpeas.

3. Stir in soy sauce or tamari and cook until veggies are tender.

4. Serve over cooked brown rice.

5. Quinoa Stuffed Bell Peppers

Ingredients:

- Bell peppers, halved and seeds removed

- 1 cup cooked quinoa

- Lean ground turkey or tofu crumbles

- Diced tomatoes

- Onion and garlic, minced

- Italian seasoning

- Salt and pepper to taste

Preparation:

1. Preheat the oven to 375°F (190°C).

2. Sauté onion and garlic, then add ground turkey or tofu crumbles.

3. Mix in diced tomatoes, cooked quinoa, and seasonings.

4. Stuff the bell pepper halves with the mixture and bake until the peppers are tender.

6. Tuna Salad Lettuce Wraps

Ingredients:

- Canned tuna (in water), drained

- Diced celery and red onion

- Greek yogurt or avocado mayo

- Dijon mustard

- Fresh lemon juice

- Lettuce leaves (romaine, butterhead)

Preparation:

1. In a bowl, mix tuna, diced celery, red onion, Greek yogurt or avocado mayo, Dijon mustard, and lemon juice.

2. Spoon the tuna salad into lettuce leaves to create wraps.

7. Mediterranean Quinoa Bowl

Ingredients:

- 1 cup cooked quinoa

- Cucumber, diced

- Cherry tomatoes, halved

- Kalamata olives, sliced

- Feta cheese, crumbled

- Fresh parsley, chopped

- Lemon vinaigrette dressing

Preparation:

1. Combine cooked quinoa, cucumber, cherry tomatoes, olives, and feta cheese.

2. Drizzle with lemon vinaigrette dressing and sprinkle with fresh parsley.

8. Zucchini Noodles with Pesto and Cherry Tomatoes

Ingredients:

- Zucchini spiralized into noodles

- Fresh basil pesto

- Cherry tomatoes, halved

- Pine nuts

- Grated Parmesan cheese

Preparation:

1. Sauté zucchini noodles until tender.

2. Toss with fresh basil pesto and top with cherry tomatoes, pine nuts, and grated Parmesan.

9. Quinoa and Black Bean Salad

Ingredients:

- 1 cup cooked quinoa

- Black beans drained and rinsed

- Bell peppers, diced

- Red onion, finely chopped

- Corn kernels (cooked or canned)

- Lime juice and zest

- Fresh cilantro, chopped

Preparation:

1. Mix cooked quinoa, black beans, bell peppers, red onion, and corn.

2. Drizzle with lime juice and zest, and garnish with fresh cilantro.

10. Grilled Veggie Wrap

Ingredients:

- Whole-grain wrap or tortilla

- Grilled vegetables (zucchini, bell peppers, eggplant)

- Hummus or Greek yogurt tzatziki

- Spinach or mixed greens

Preparation:

1. Spread hummus or tzatziki on the wrap.

2. Layer with grilled vegetables and spinach or mixed greens.

3. Roll up the wrap and enjoy a flavorful lunch.

The Galveston Diet lunch meal plan emphasizes nutrient-dense, balanced, and flavorful options that align with the principles of hormonal balance and overall wellness. By incorporating these recipes into your lunchtime routine, you provide your body with essential nutrients while promoting vitality and well-being. Customize these recipes to suit your taste preferences and dietary needs, and enjoy the benefits of a nourishing and satisfying lunch that supports your health goals.

Chapter 6

The Galveston Diet Meal Plan For Dinner

The Galveston Diet dinner meal plan emphasizes nourishing and balanced options that promote hormonal balance and overall well-being. By focusing on lean proteins, fiber-rich carbohydrates, healthy fats, and a variety of vegetables, these dinner recipes provide a satisfying and health-conscious way to end the day.

1. Baked Lemon Herb Chicken with Roasted Vegetables

Ingredients:

- 4 boneless, skinless chicken breasts

- Lemon juice and zest

- Fresh herbs (rosemary, thyme)

- Mixed vegetables (carrots, broccoli, bell peppers)

- Olive oil

- Salt and pepper to taste

Preparation:

1. Preheat the oven to 375°F (190°C).

2. Marinate chicken in lemon juice, zest, herbs, salt, and pepper.

3. Bake chicken and roast mixed vegetables with olive oil until tender.

2. Seared Salmon with Steamed Asparagus and Quinoa

Ingredients

- 4 salmon fillets

- Asparagus spears, trimmed

- 1 cup cooked quinoa

- Lemon juice

- Fresh dill

- Salt and pepper to taste

Preparation:

1. Season salmon with salt and pepper, and sear in a skillet.

2. Steam asparagus, squeeze lemon juice, and sprinkle with fresh dill.

3. Serve salmon and asparagus over quinoa, garnished with more dill.

3. Turkey and Vegetable Stir-Fry

Ingredients:

- Lean ground turkey

- Mixed vegetables (bell peppers, snap peas, carrots)

- Low-sodium soy sauce or tamari

- Garlic and ginger, minced

- Sesame oil

- Cooked brown rice

Preparation:

1. Sauté garlic and ginger in sesame oil.

2. Add ground turkey and cook until browned.

3. Stir in mixed vegetables and soy sauce, and cook until tender.

4. Serve over cooked brown rice.

4. Quinoa-Stuffed Portobello Mushrooms

Ingredients:

- Portobello mushroom caps

- 1 cup cooked quinoa

- Spinach, chopped

- Sun-dried tomatoes, chopped

- Red onion, diced

- Feta cheese

- Olive oil

- Salt and pepper to taste

Preparation:

1. Preheat the oven to 375°F (190°C).

2. Brush mushroom caps with olive oil, and roast until tender.

3. Mix quinoa, spinach, tomatoes, onion, feta, salt, and pepper.

4. Stuff mushrooms with the quinoa mixture and bake until heated through.

5. Vegetable and Chickpea Curry

Ingredients:

- Mixed vegetables (cauliflower, carrots, bell peppers)

- Cooked chickpeas

- Curry paste or powder

- Coconut milk

- Onion and garlic, minced

- Fresh cilantro, chopped

- Cooked brown rice

Preparation:

1. Sauté onion and garlic, add curry paste/powder, and mixed vegetables.

2. Stir in chickpeas and coconut milk, and simmer until veggies are tender.

3. Serve over cooked brown rice, garnished with fresh cilantro.

6. Grilled Tofu and Broccoli with Quinoa

Ingredients:

- Firm tofu, sliced

- Broccoli florets

- Low-sodium soy sauce or tamari

- Garlic, minced

- Sesame oil

- Cooked quinoa

Preparation:

1. Marinate tofu in soy sauce, garlic, and sesame oil.

2. Grill tofu and steam broccoli until tender.

3. Serve tofu and broccoli over quinoa.

7. Mediterranean Baked Cod with Greek Salad

Ingredients:

- Cod fillets

- Lemon juice and zest

- Fresh oregano

- Cherry tomatoes, halved

- Cucumber, diced

- Red onion, thinly sliced

- Kalamata olives, sliced

- Feta cheese

- Olive oil

- Salt and pepper to taste

Preparation:

1. Preheat the oven to 375°F (190°C).

2. Marinate cod with lemon, oregano, salt, and pepper.

3. Bake cod and prepare a Greek salad with tomatoes, cucumber, onion, olives, feta, and olive oil.

8. Zucchini and Tomato Stuffed Bell Peppers

Ingredients:

- Bell peppers, halved and seeds removed

- Zucchini diced

- Cherry tomatoes, halved

- Red onion, finely chopped

- Fresh basil, chopped

- Olive oil

- Salt and pepper to taste

Preparation:

1. Preheat the oven to 375°F (190°C).

2. Sauté zucchini, tomatoes, and onion, mix with fresh basil, salt, and pepper.

3. Stuff bell pepper halves with the mixture and bake until the peppers are tender.

9. Spaghetti Squash with Turkey Meatballs and Marinara

Ingredients:

- Spaghetti squash

- Lean ground turkey

- Whole-grain breadcrumbs

- Garlic and onion, minced

- Italian seasoning

- Low-sodium marinara sauce

Preparation:

1. Preheat the oven to 375°F (190°C).

2. Roast spaghetti squash, scrape out the strands.

3. Mix ground turkey, breadcrumbs, garlic, onion, and seasoning, and form into meatballs.

4. Bake meatballs and serve over spaghetti squash with marinara sauce.

10. Balsamic Glazed Vegetable Skewers with Quinoa

Ingredients:

- Mixed vegetables (zucchini, bell peppers, red onion)

- Balsamic vinegar

- Olive oil

- Fresh rosemary

- Cooked quinoa

Preparation:

1. Heat up the grill or oven to a medium-high temperature in advance.

2. Thread vegetables onto skewers, brush with balsamic vinegar, olive oil, and rosemary.

3. Grill or roast skewers until vegetables are charred and tender.

4. Serve over cooked quinoa.

The Galveston Diet dinner meal plan provides a wide array of satisfying and nutrient-rich options that align with the principles of hormone balance and overall wellness. These recipes allow you to enjoy flavorful, well-balanced dinners that support your health goals and contribute to a sense of vitality. Customize these recipes to suit your individual preferences and dietary needs, and relish in the benefits of a nourishing and delicious dinner routine.

Chapter 7

Exercise and Motion for Optimal Well-being

The threads of exercise and motion are woven with profound significance, creating a vibrant canvas of optimal well-being. Beyond the confines of physical activity, the art of movement resonates across the dimensions of physical health, mental acuity, emotional balance, and spiritual alignment. In this chapter, we embark on a journey through the intricate pathways of exercise and motion, uncovering their multifaceted impact on the body, mind, and spirit, and illuminating the strategies to integrate them seamlessly into the tapestry of our lives.

The Symphony of Physical Well-being

At the heart of exercise and motion lies a symphony of physical benefits that harmonize the body's intricate systems. Physical well-being is a dynamic interplay of strength, flexibility, cardiovascular health, and metabolic efficiency.

Strengthening Muscles and Bones: Engaging in regular physical activity nourishes the body's musculoskeletal system, fostering the growth and maintenance of lean muscle mass and promoting bone density. Weight-bearing exercises, resistance training, and even activities like yoga and Pilates stimulate muscle fibers and bones, creating a fortress of physical resilience.

Cardiovascular Brilliance: The cardiovascular system, a symphony of vessels and chambers, thrives under the influence of exercise. Aerobic activities, such as running, swimming, and cycling, challenge the heart to pump blood efficiently, strengthening its muscle and enhancing its ability to deliver oxygen and nutrients to tissues.

Regular cardio workouts lower blood pressure, reduce the risk of heart disease and improve overall cardiovascular health.

Metabolic Magic: The dance of exercise and motion orchestrates metabolic magic within the body. Physical activity revs up the metabolism, enhancing the body's ability to burn calories and maintain a healthy weight. Moreover, regular exercise contributes to better insulin sensitivity, a cornerstone in diabetes prevention and management.

Mental Clarity and Cognitive Brilliance

The effects of exercise extend beyond the realm of the physical, permeating the corridors of mental clarity and cognitive brilliance. Engaging in movement sparks a symphony of neurochemical reactions that enhance cognitive function and mental well-being.

Neurotransmitters and Mood Elevation: The brain becomes a theater of transformation during exercise, releasing a cascade of neurotransmitters that elevate mood and alleviate stress. Endorphins, commonly referred to as the body's natural pain relievers, trigger sensations of euphoria and calmness. Serotonin, the mood-regulating neurotransmitter, flourishes under the influence of physical activity, fostering emotional balance.

Cognitive Enhancement and Neuroplasticity: The mind undergoes a process of cognitive refinement through exercise. Physical activity enhances blood flow to the brain, nourishing brain cells and promoting neuroplasticity—the brain's ability to adapt and rewire itself. This translates to improved memory, enhanced cognitive function, and reduced risk of cognitive decline.

Emotional Equilibrium and Stress Resilience

In the realm of emotional well-being, exercise, and motion unfurls a tapestry of resilience, equipping individuals with the tools to navigate the ebb and flow of emotions with grace.

Stress-Relieving Symphony: Movement acts as a powerful counterbalance to the stressors of modern life. Engaging in physical activity prompts the release of stress hormones, allowing the body to recalibrate and return to a state of equilibrium. The rhythmic flow of motion provides a cathartic outlet for pent-up tension, fostering emotional well-being.

Anxiety Reduction and Emotional Serenity: The melodies of exercise extend their soothing touch to anxiety reduction. Regular physical activity reduces the levels of anxiety-inducing chemicals in the brain, creating a shield of emotional serenity. The meditative aspects of activities like yoga and tai chi further enhance this effect, allowing individuals to cultivate mindfulness and find solace amidst life's challenges.

The Dance of Sleep and Renewal

As the sun sets and darkness envelops the world, the role of exercise and motion in sleep quality comes to the forefront. The choreography of physical activity and restful sleep weaves a tapestry of renewal that enhances overall well-being.

Sleep Induction and Quality: The rhythm of movement harmonizes with the rhythm of sleep, influencing sleep induction and quality. Engaging in regular physical activity helps regulate circadian rhythms, promoting a balanced sleep-wake cycle. The synergy between exercise and sleep goes beyond the duration of slumber, extending to the realm of sleep quality. Individuals who embrace movement often experience deeper and more restorative sleep.

Mindful Movement and Sleep Harmony: The harmony between exercise and sleep quality is amplified when mindful movement takes center stage. Activities like gentle stretching, yoga, and meditation become the prelude to sleep, easing the transition from wakefulness to rest. These practices calm the mind, relax the body, and set the stage for a peaceful night's sleep.

The Symphony of Integration: Strategies for Embracing Exercise and Motion:

Embarking on a journey of exercise and motion is a testament to embracing the symphony of integration—aligning physical, mental, and emotional dimensions for optimal well-being. The following strategies guide this harmonious integration:

Personalized Movement: Discover activities that resonate with your preferences and align with your physical condition. Embrace activities that bring joy, whether it's dancing, hiking, swimming, or practicing martial arts.

Consistency and Routine: Establishing a consistent exercise routine creates a foundation for well-being. Aim for regularity in your activities, even if it means starting with shorter durations. Consistency nurtures a sustainable and long-lasting relationship with movement.

Variety and Playfulness: Embrace the art of variety by incorporating diverse exercises into your routine. Balance cardiovascular workouts with strength training, flexibility exercises, and mindful practices that foster holistic well-being.

Mindful Movement: Cultivate mindfulness in every step of your journey. Whether it's a brisk walk in nature, a serene yoga session, or a vigorous workout, infuse each moment with mindfulness, immersing yourself fully in the experience.

Holistic Hydration and Nutrition: Hydration and nutrition form the canvas upon which the symphony of exercise is painted. Prioritize nourishing foods that provide energy and support muscle recovery. Stay hydrated to optimize performance and promote overall well-being.

Progressive Challenges: As you traverse the path of exercise and motion, set progressive challenges that propel you forward. Gradually increase the intensity, duration, and complexity of your activities to continually challenge and nourish your body and mind.

Mind-Body Fusion: Embrace the profound connection between mind and body. Engage in activities that synchronize movement with breath, cultivating a sense of unity between physical action and inner awareness.

Rest and Recovery: Honor the importance of rest and recovery as integral components of the symphony of movement. Allow your body the time it needs to rejuvenate and heal, ensuring a balanced approach to well-being.

Exercise and motion compose a vibrant and harmonious melody that reverberates across the dimensions of well-being. The art of movement becomes a canvas upon which physical vitality, mental clarity, emotional balance, and spiritual alignment are painted. By embracing exercise as a transformative journey, we unleash the power of movement to uplift and enrich every facet of our existence. As we dance through life with intention, guided by the rhythms of our bodies and the melodies of our hearts, we compose a symphony of vitality, joy, and optimal well-being.

Chapter 8

Stress Control and Enhancing Sleep Quality

Stress has evolved into an almost ever-present companion for numerous individuals. The demands of work, family, and personal aspirations create a complex symphony of responsibilities that can leave individuals feeling overwhelmed and fatigued. However, stress need not be an unconquerable adversary; it can be tamed and managed through intentional practices that restore equilibrium. In parallel, the pursuit of quality sleep becomes paramount, as it serves as the foundation upon which the pillars of well-being stand. In this exploration, we delve into the art of stress control and the enhancement of sleep quality, uncovering the profound impact of these practices on physical health, mental clarity, and emotional serenity.

Stress Control

Stress, often dubbed the "silent killer," permeates every aspect of existence, affecting individuals physically, mentally, and emotionally. Left unchecked, chronic stress can pave the way for a host of ailments, ranging from cardiovascular disorders to anxiety and depression. However, the human spirit is remarkably resilient, and strategies for stress control empower individuals to navigate life's tumultuous waters with grace and resilience.

Mindfulness and Meditation: At the heart of stress control lies the art of mindfulness and meditation. These practices offer a refuge from the chaos, inviting individuals to anchor themselves in the present moment. Mindfulness encourages the cultivation of awareness, allowing thoughts and emotions to flow without judgment. Meditation, on the other hand, provides a sanctuary for the mind, fostering a sense of calm and introspection. Regular practice of mindfulness and meditation equips individuals with tools to manage stress by offering a space for reflection, self-compassion, and detachment from the whirlwind of daily life.

Breathwork and Relaxation Techniques: The breath, a constant life companion, becomes a powerful ally in the quest for stress control. Breathwork techniques, such as deep breathing and diaphragmatic breathing, activate the body's relaxation response, triggering a cascade of physiological changes that counteract stress. These techniques serve as immediate interventions during moments of stress, restoring a sense of calm and equilibrium. Incorporating relaxation techniques, such as progressive muscle relaxation and guided imagery, further enhances stress reduction by guiding individuals into states of deep relaxation and mental clarity.

Physical Activity as Stress Relief: The symbiotic relationship between the body and mind is exemplified through the stress-reducing effects of physical activity. Engaging in regular exercise, whether through brisk walks, invigorating runs, or the practice of yoga, releases endorphins, commonly referred to as "feel-good" hormones. These endorphins act as natural stress relievers, soothing the mind and promoting emotional well-being. Moreover, physical activity serves as a channel for releasing pent-up tension and anxiety, providing an outlet for the accumulation of daily stressors.

Cultivating Resilience and Healthy Coping Mechanisms: Beyond specific practices, the cultivation of resilience and healthy coping mechanisms form the bedrock of stress control. Adopting a growth mindset, reframing challenges as opportunities, and nurturing self-compassion are powerful ways to build resilience in the face of stress. Additionally, cultivating hobbies, connecting with loved ones, and engaging in creative expression offer avenues for healthy emotional release and contribute to a well-rounded approach to stress management.

Enhancing Sleep Quality

As the sun sets and darkness envelops the world, sleep emerges as a vital companion, inviting the body and mind into a state of rejuvenation. Quality sleep is not a luxury but a physiological necessity that underpins physical vitality, cognitive sharpness, and emotional balance. Enhancing sleep quality requires the implementation of practices that honor the body's natural rhythms and create a sanctuary for rest.

Prioritizing Sleep Hygiene: The foundation of enhancing sleep quality lies in the establishment of sound sleep hygiene practices. This entails creating a sleep-conducive environment that promotes relaxation and tranquility.

Dimming lights, limiting screen time before bed, and ensuring a comfortable mattress and pillows are crucial steps in setting the stage for restful slumber. Additionally, establishing a consistent sleep schedule, where waking and sleeping times remain relatively constant, supports the body's internal clock and aids in achieving restorative sleep.

Creating a Soothing Bedtime Ritual: A soothing bedtime ritual serves as a bridge between the activities of the day and the embrace of sleep. Engaging in calming practices such as reading, journaling, or sipping herbal tea can signal to the body that it is time to unwind. The act of disconnecting from digital devices and engaging in mindful activities fosters relaxation, allowing the mind to transition from the busyness of the day to a state of quiet contemplation.

Nutrition and Sleep: The interplay between nutrition and sleep is profound, as dietary choices can impact sleep quality. Consuming caffeine and heavy, rich foods close to bedtime can disrupt sleep patterns. Conversely, opting for sleep-enhancing foods like whole grains, lean proteins, and foods rich in tryptophan (an amino acid precursor to serotonin) can promote better sleep. Hydration also plays a role; ensuring adequate water intake throughout the day can prevent nighttime awakenings due to thirst.

Stress Reduction for Better Sleep: The synergy between stress control and sleep quality is a reciprocal one. Managing stress through mindfulness, relaxation, and physical activity can positively influence sleep by reducing the mind's propensity to race and the body's release of stress hormones. As stress levels decrease, the likelihood of falling into restorative sleep increases, allowing individuals to wake up feeling refreshed and rejuvenated.

Stress control and the enhancement of sleep quality stand as two interconnected pillars of well-being that nurture harmony within the complex symphony of life. The practices and strategies explored in this journey offer avenues for individuals to navigate the challenges of modern existence with grace and resilience. By embracing mindfulness, meditation, breathwork, and physical activity, individuals harness the tools to tame stress's unruly waves and restore equilibrium to the mind and body. Simultaneously, the art of sleep enhancement, encompassing sleep hygiene, bedtime rituals, nutrition, and stress reduction, creates a haven for restful slumber, allowing the body and mind to dance in the rhythm of replenishment. As we weave these practices into the fabric of our lives, we embark on a journey of holistic well-being, marked by vitality, clarity, and emotional serenity. In the delicate dance between stress control and sleep enhancement, we discover the art of living in harmony amidst the chaos of existence.

Chapter 9

Menopause and the Galveston Diet Strategy

The journey of womanhood is a remarkable tapestry woven with various stages, each marked by unique physical and hormonal changes. One of the most significant transitions in a woman's life is menopause, a natural process signifying the end of reproductive years. As the body undergoes intricate hormonal shifts, it is crucial to approach this phase with mindfulness and empowerment. The Galveston Diet Strategy, an innovative approach to nutrition and well-being, offers a guiding light through the labyrinth of menopause, providing insights and strategies to navigate this transformative journey with grace and vitality.

Menopause: An Intricate Transformation

Menopause is a natural biological event that occurs when a woman's menstrual cycle ceases, typically around the age of 45 to 55. This transition is marked by a decrease in the production of estrogen and progesterone, leading to various physical and emotional changes. Common symptoms of menopause include hot flashes, night sweats, mood fluctuations, weight gain, and changes in bone density.

The Galveston Diet Strategy: A Holistic Approach

The Galveston Diet Strategy emerges as a beacon of hope, offering a holistic approach to nutrition, hormonal balance, and overall well-being. Rooted in scientific research and designed by experts, this strategy recognizes the importance of nourishing the body with nutrient-dense foods that support hormonal harmony and mitigate the challenges of menopause.

Balancing Hormones through Nutrition

The Galveston Diet Strategy focuses on optimizing hormone levels through strategic food choices. It emphasizes the consumption of whole foods, rich in essential nutrients that support hormonal balance. These foods include lean proteins, healthy fats, fiber-rich carbohydrates, and a variety of fruits and vegetables. By fueling the body with these nutrient-dense options, women can help alleviate the hormonal imbalances that often accompany menopause.

Mitigating Weight Gain and Supporting Metabolism

Weight gain is a common concern during menopause due to hormonal fluctuations and changes in metabolism. The Galveston Diet Strategy addresses this challenge by advocating for balanced and portion-controlled meals. By incorporating lean proteins, such as poultry, fish, and plant-based sources, along with fiber-rich carbohydrates and healthy fats, women can stabilize blood sugar levels and support a healthy metabolism. This strategy also encourages mindful eating and emphasizes the importance of staying hydrated.

Reducing Inflammation and Supporting Bone Health

Inflammation and bone health are vital considerations during menopause. The Galveston Diet Strategy promotes anti-inflammatory foods, such as leafy greens, berries, and fatty fish rich in omega-3 fatty acids. These foods help reduce inflammation, which can contribute to a range of health issues. Additionally, the strategy emphasizes the importance of calcium and vitamin D-rich foods, essential for maintaining strong and healthy bones as women age.

Managing Mood and Emotional Well-being

The emotional rollercoaster often associated with menopause is not disregarded by the Galveston Diet Strategy. It underscores the significance of nutrient-rich foods that support brain health and emotional well-being. Omega-3 fatty acids, found in foods like salmon, walnuts, and flaxseeds, are particularly beneficial for mood stabilization and cognitive function. The strategy also advocates for the consumption of complex carbohydrates, which help regulate serotonin levels and promote a positive mood.

Incorporating Phytoestrogens and Nutrient-Rich Superfoods

Phytoestrogens, plant-based compounds that mimic estrogen in the body, play a role in mitigating the hormonal changes of menopause. The Galveston Diet Strategy encourages the inclusion of phytoestrogen-rich foods, such as soy, flaxseeds, and legumes. These foods can help alleviate some of the symptoms of hormonal imbalance and promote overall well-being.

Strategies for Implementation and Lifestyle Integration

The Galveston Diet Strategy is not merely a set of dietary guidelines; it is a comprehensive lifestyle approach that supports women in their journey through menopause. For successful integration of this approach, take into account the following:

Educate Yourself: Take the time to understand the principles and guidelines of the Galveston Diet Strategy. Knowledge empowers you to make informed choices that align with your health goals.

Plan Meals Thoughtfully: Plan and prepare balanced meals that incorporate a variety of nutrient-dense foods. Emphasize lean proteins, fiber-rich carbohydrates, healthy fats, and a rainbow of fruits and vegetables.

Practice Mindful Eating: Engage in mindful eating practices that promote awareness and enjoyment of your meals. Take your time while chewing, relish the tastes, and remain mindful of your body's signals of hunger and fullness.

Stay Hydrated: Hydration is essential for overall well-being. Drink an adequate amount of water throughout the day to support digestion, metabolism, and hormonal balance.

Prioritize Physical Activity: Regular exercise complements the Galveston Diet Strategy by promoting weight management, bone health, and emotional well-being. Engage in activities you enjoy, whether it's walking, dancing, yoga, or strength training.

Manage Stress: Menopause can be a stressful time, but stress management is crucial for hormonal balance. Incorporate relaxation techniques such as deep breathing, meditation, and mindfulness to alleviate stress and promote emotional equilibrium.

Seek Professional Guidance: Consult a healthcare professional or registered dietitian before making significant dietary changes, especially during menopause. They have the ability to offer tailored advice depending on your specific requirements and health condition.

The Galveston Diet Strategy serves as a compass, guiding women through the transformative landscape of menopause with wisdom, empowerment, and nutritional nourishment. By embracing this holistic approach to well-being, women can navigate the hormonal transitions of menopause with grace, vitality, and a renewed sense of self. As they embark on this journey of transformation, they harness the power of nutrition, movement, and self-care, cultivating a radiant and empowered life beyond menopause.

Chapter 10

Sustained Weight Management with the Galveston Diet

The quest for sustained weight management can often feel like an elusive and challenging endeavor. However, the Galveston Diet emerges as a refreshing beacon of hope, offering a comprehensive and science-based approach to weight management that extends beyond short-term solutions. Rooted in the principles of nutrition, hormonal balance, and holistic well-being, the Galveston Diet provides a roadmap to achieve and maintain a healthy weight, empowering individuals to embark on a transformative journey towards lifelong wellness.

Understanding Sustained Weight Management

Sustained weight management goes beyond the numbers on a scale; it encompasses a holistic approach to health and well-being. It involves creating a balanced and sustainable lifestyle that supports both physical and emotional vitality. While weight loss may be an initial goal, the ultimate aspiration is to achieve a state of equilibrium where the body functions optimally, energy levels are vibrant, and overall wellness thrives.

The Galveston Diet

The Galveston Diet is not a fleeting trend; it is a thoughtful and evidence-based strategy that focuses on nurturing the body, regulating hormones, and embracing a mindful approach to nutrition. This approach empowers individuals to break free from the cycle of yo-yo dieting and embark on a transformative journey toward sustained weight management.

Hormonal Harmony and Weight Regulation

One of the cornerstones of the Galveston Diet is its emphasis on hormonal balance. Hormones play a pivotal role in weight regulation, metabolism, and overall well-being. The Galveston Diet recognizes the intricate interplay between hormones, particularly insulin, and cortisol, and their impact on weight management. By making strategic food choices that stabilize blood sugar levels and reduce inflammation, individuals can promote hormonal harmony and create an environment conducive to sustained weight management.

Balancing Macronutrients for Optimal Energy

The Galveston Diet emphasizes the importance of balanced macronutrients—proteins, carbohydrates, and fats—to fuel the body and sustain energy levels. Lean proteins provide the building blocks for muscle growth and repair, while healthy fats support satiety and cognitive function. Fiber-rich carbohydrates provide sustained energy and stabilize blood sugar levels. By crafting meals that incorporate a balance of these macronutrients, individuals can experience prolonged satiety, reduced cravings, and enhanced energy throughout the day.

Mindful Eating for Long-Term Success

Mindful eating is a cornerstone of the Galveston Diet, promoting a conscious and intentional relationship with food. Mindful eating encourages individuals to listen to their bodies hunger and fullness cues, savor the flavors of each bite, and cultivate a deep awareness of the eating experience. This practice fosters a sense of satisfaction and prevents overeating, contributing to sustained weight management.

Incorporating Nutrient-Dense Foods

The Galveston Diet prioritizes nutrient-dense foods that nourish the body and support overall health. These foods include a rich variety of fruits, vegetables, whole grains, lean proteins, and healthy fats. Nutrient-dense foods provide essential vitamins, minerals, and antioxidants that promote cellular health, immune function, and vitality. By incorporating these foods into daily meals, individuals not only support their weight management goals but also enhance their overall well-being.

Strategies for Sustainable Implementation

Achieving and maintaining sustained weight management through the Galveston Diet involves a mindful and strategic approach. Consider the following strategies to integrate the Galveston Diet principles into your lifestyle:

Educate Yourself: Take the time to understand the core principles and guidelines of the Galveston Diet. Knowledge empowers you to make informed choices that align with your health goals.

Plan Balanced Meals: Craft-balanced meals that incorporate a variety of nutrient-dense foods. Focus on portion control, and ensure that each meal includes lean proteins, fiber-rich carbohydrates, and healthy fats.

Physical Activity: Combine the Galveston Diet with regular physical activity to enhance weight management and promote overall fitness. Engage in activities you enjoy, whether it's brisk walking, dancing, yoga, or strength training.

Make sleep a priority: High-quality sleep plays a critical role in weight management and hormonal equilibrium. Create a sleep-conducive environment, establish a consistent sleep routine, and prioritize restful slumber.

Mind-Body Connection: Cultivate a strong mind-body connection by practicing stress-reduction techniques such as deep breathing, meditation, and yoga. Managing stress supports hormonal balance and emotional well-being.

Consistency and Patience: Sustained weight management is a journey that requires consistency and patience. Embrace gradual progress, celebrate small victories, and stay committed to your long-term goals.

The Galveston Diet serves as a compass guiding individuals toward sustained weight management and lifelong wellness. By integrating the principles of hormonal balance, mindful eating, and nutrient-dense foods, individuals can embark on a transformative journey that transcends fleeting weight loss trends. The Galveston Diet empowers individuals to create a harmonious relationship with their bodies, nurturing vitality, and embracing a balanced and vibrant life. As individuals embrace the Galveston Diet as a way of life, they unlock the potential for sustained weight management, enhanced well-being, and a future marked by vitality and holistic health.